Making Disabled Life Easier

Eva Sessions' Guide to Adjusting and Making the Most of Living with a Disability

Eva Sessions

Joan Levenson Bruni

Contents

Foreword

This book is written in the voice of my mother, Eva Sessions. It was her idea to write this book, and it is her story. She lost her eyesight suddenly due to an illness, and went from fully functioning to having a significant disability in a matter of days. To her credit, my mother made the best of an unfortunate situation. She worked at making her life as comfortable and fulfilling as she could, and along the way she learned a lot about living with a disability.

My mother wanted to write this book to share her knowledge with others who might be facing similar circumstances. She began dictating her thoughts into a digital recorder, and then one of her caregivers, the ever-patient Chantal Zeitler, transcribed them for her. When I read the transcriptions, I realized that my mother had good ideas, but her writing was more like an office procedure manual, which was not surprising because my mother's career encompassed administrative positions in nursing and public health.

So, I offered to rewrite it for her as a book. Needless to say, I had underestimated the time commitment involved, so my work on the book progressed very slowly. Much too slowly for my mother, who wanted to see it finished while she was still alive. I tried to work on it as much as I could, but my commitments as a wife and the mother of a young son involved in numerous sports, and my part-time job as a post-doctoral psychotherapist, did not leave me with a lot of spare time. Unfortunately, my mother died before the book was completed. I had promised her I would finish it, so I continued to work on it, and now it is done.

This book is not a comprehensive guide to living with a disability, nor is it intended to be. It is one woman's story and her suggestions about how to go on living when you have a disability. My mother's story is noteworthy, however, because of how well she handled her sudden loss and was able to go on with her life. After she went blind, people told her she should sue the doctors who failed to diagnose her illness in time to save her sight. She consulted with an attorney, but he told her that because she had not exhibited the most common symptoms, the doctors likely would not be found negligent, and thus she did not have a case. The attorney also told me privately that, in researching my mother's illness, he found that most victims died within a year after losing their sight. The fact that my mother lived another five years, and was able to make the most of that time is a testament to her indomitable spirit. My mother was indeed a remarkable woman.

I love you, Mom. Here is your book. I finally finished it.

Joan Levenson Bruni

Acknowledgements

Many people helped to make this book a reality. First, Dr. Anne Carter, audiologist, gave me the initial encouragement to compile these suggestions into a book that could be helpful to others. In addition, she put my transcribed words into a format in which they could be worked with more easily, and she provided information about talking to an individual with a hearing impairment. My dear friend, Nancy Haak, and her daughter, Holly Hines, also encouraged me, and helped to focus my broad range of ideas into a manageable outline. My wonderful caregiver and delightful friend, Chantal Zeitler, patiently transcribed my dictations and then reread them back to me, over and over again. And finally, my daughter Joan Bruni, took those transcribed dictations and wrote this book for me. Others who assisted in the preparation of this book include my dear longtime friend, Cathy Frasca, and newer friends, Judy Walsh, BN, RN., Beth Hughes, RN., Cecilia Leth, PT, Sonia Geiger, Tom Talbot, Sharon Spesak, and Kathleen Stowe. I thank all of you from the bottom of my heart!

Eva Sessions

Introduction

On Thursday, April 5th, 2007, I woke up blind.

That sentence sounds like the plot for an episode of <u>The Twilight Zone</u>, or one of those medical mystery dramas on TV. It certainly does not sound like something I would have expected to happen to me – a healthy, active, and very independent 81-year-old woman enjoying her retirement in South Florida. But it did.

Two days earlier, I had driven myself to an eye specialist because I was seeing a spot in front of my right eye. He told me to go to the hospital immediately for treatment of temporal arteritis, a disease I had never heard of prior to that day. Temporal arteritis is an inflammation of the temporal arteries. It can choke off the oxygen supply to the optic nerve, leading to blindness. The cause is uncertain, but it affects older adults. It is rare in those under 50, and the incidence increases in those over 80. The main symptom is a severe headache, which I never had. Looking back, I had more subtle symptoms – vague neck and head pain, which I had attributed to the sinus problems and fibromyalgia I had dealt with for years.

Following the doctor's directions, I checked myself into the local hospital that afternoon. I received high doses of steroids to try to reduce the inflammation, but unfortunately the treatment had begun too late. By Thursday morning, I had lost all the vision in my right eye and 95% of the vision in my left eye. The doctors told me that blindness caused by temporal arteritis is almost never reversible. For the rest of my life, I would be almost completely blind. The active, independent life I had been living a week earlier was gone.

As anyone who has experienced a sudden disability can tell you, adjusting to life with a disability is not easy, especially when you live alone. I have been widowed and divorced, so like many women of my age, I have no spouse to take care of me. I have one child, a daughter living up north in Pittsburgh, Pennsylvania, but she has a young child and a husband who owns a restaurant and works 70-75 hours per week, so it is not feasible for her to come to Florida to take care of me. She and her husband wanted me to come live with them, but I left those cold winters behind and have no interest in experiencing them again. Besides, I love my cozy two-bedroom condominium with its beautiful view of the sun setting over the Gulf of Mexico. I have lived here for more than twenty-five years and know it better than the back of my hand. If there is anywhere I want to live as a blind person, it is in my own condo. Even though I may never see those sunsets again, at least I know they are there, and I can experience them again in my mind.

I am not a rich woman, but my late husband's Coast Guard survivors' benefits and the money he left me have given me the means to hire caregivers so I can remain in my own home. I realize many people will not be able to hire caregivers, but I have included a section about hiring caregivers in this book. My experiences with caregivers and the agencies that provide them have ranged from excellent to abysmal, and I am hoping that what I have learned from those experiences can help other disabled people avoid the abysmal part!

I now have some wonderful caregivers, and it has been four years since I lost my eyesight. During that time, and throughout the ordeal of sudden blindness and creating a new life for myself, I have been doing a lot of learning about how to make things easier for myself. I have learned on my own through trial and error, and I have learned from professionals such as doctors, nurses, physical therapists and occupational therapists. The professionals taught me little tricks or new ways of doing things that can make living with a handicap less of a daily struggle.

This learning was often happenstance. A professional would be surprised that no one had shown me a certain way to do something, or I would stumble upon a gadget or system that would solve a minor but irritating problem, or even a major problem. And with each instance of learning, I would think, "I wish I had known this earlier!" As those "I wish I had known this earlier!" moments piled up, I realized that, while I could not go back and make my own initial experience with disabled life easier, I could help someone else adjust to a sudden loss of ability. Thus, the idea for this book was born. I decided to compile everything that I had learned into a book that could make life easier, and increase comfort and independence, for people with disabilities and their caregivers.

In addition, I have been doing a lot of teaching since I became handicapped – teaching my caregivers and some of the health care providers I have encountered. My professional background is in nursing and public health (I have masters' degrees in both those fields), and I learned nursing back in the days when proper bedside care was taught and valued. Accordingly, I am frequently surprised by how many health care professionals and paraprofessionals are unaware of simple techniques and procedures that can increase a patient's comfort, and even more important, prevent additional injury or illness. Therefore, this book also contains some things that I have had to teach since I became disabled.

In summary, this book is intended for someone who is dealing with a handicap or disability, especially someone who has suddenly become disabled, and also to anyone who is providing care to someone with a disability. It is based on my own experience, and as such, it is not intended to be exhaustive or all-encompassing. It is just the information I know and have learned since I lost my eyesight, and wish I had known sooner. If one person finds that some of this information makes it easier to live with a disability, my efforts will have been worthwhile.

One

Guiding Stars to Keep Your Life on Course

Many people recoil from the idea of adding more rules to their lives. The word "rule" sounds so rigid and no fun at all, like the second grade teacher who prohibits talking in class or running in the halls. If asked whether they would like to add more rules to their lives, most people would probably say, "No!" - Especially those people who have disabilities. A disability feels limiting enough – why add more limits to their lives?

Yet we all know that rules are useful. They provide structure and keep things from spiraling out of control. Imagine a second-grade classroom without any rules! Rules help to keep us safe, and also keep us from going too far off course, which is why I have chosen to begin this book by presenting my three main rules for living with a disability.

These three rules have helped me to move forward toward my goal of a full and satisfying life, and have helped me to avoid getting stuck in a mire of increasing disability and depression. But since the word "rule" itself might sound too depressing to some people, I'll call them "guiding stars" instead.

Guiding Star #1:
Safety first! Avoid Another Disability!

Focusing on safety might sound unnecessary to someone who is recently disabled: "Of course I'm going to be safe now that I'm disabled! I've cancelled my sky-diving lessons and given away my skateboard. What more do you want me to do?"

But what many people fail to realize is that activities that were relatively safe and innocuous before a disability, often take on added risk when your body does not have the capabilities it had before. Crossing a street near the end of the "Walk" signal is not very dangerous when you can quicken your stride when the light changes. But when you are unable to move quickly, the situation can become rather dicey. Similarly, heating food in a microwave, or even walking across a room, can become risky activities if you have lost your eyesight. And while you might say, "Oh well, what's wrong with a little risk – I am already disabled anyway," you might want to consider that a serious fall or burn, or being hit by a car, could lead to increased disability, which is something most of us want to avoid.

I learned this lesson about newly dangerous activities the hard way. Unbeknownst to me, losing one's eyesight affects one's balance. (If you don't believe me, try standing on one foot for 30 seconds with your eyes open, and then again with your eyes closed!) One day, I was sitting on a kitchen stool, trying to put a heating pad on my ankle. I bent down, reached toward my ankle, and toppled headfirst onto the floor. Because of my age and my osteoporosis, that fall fractured vertebrae in my back, and was a serious setback for me, both physically and emotionally.

This guiding star is not intended to scare people with disabilities into sitting in a chair and covering themselves in bubble wrap for the rest of their lives. Instead, I use this Guiding Star to remind me to think about safety in whatever I am doing. I try not to rush, and I try to think about the safest way to do something before I attempt to do it. I also try to concentrate solely on what I am doing. Save multitasking until you are truly proficient in the activity!

Guiding Star #2:
Live as Independently as Possible, but Be Willing to Accept Help When Necessary.

My second guiding star, or rule to live by, can be a little bit tricky. While "Safety first" is pretty clear-cut with one main goal – keeping oneself safe, the second rule requires balancing two goals that seem to conflict – living independently and accepting help. In actuality, however, these two goals can work together, as I have learned from my own experience. By accepting help when I need it, I have been able to remain in my own home and maintain my independence. The key is to know when to do things on your own, and when to accept or request assistance.

When one is newly disabled, it is often tempting to go to one of two extremes – either trying to do everything on your own, notwithstanding the disability, or letting others do everything for you. People sometimes start out at the first extreme, trying to ignore or deny the disability, and then when that does not work (because they no longer have the physical ability to do certain things), they give up and go to the other extreme, becoming very dependent and wanting others to wait on them hand and foot. That dependent approach has its benefits. Being taken care of and catered to can help compensate for the losses that come with disability, and it removes the stress of trying to do things independently, which can be scary and frustrating. Ultimately, however, the dependent approach tends to backfire. The dependent person, by not even attempting to do things on his own, loses self-respect and forgoes the satisfaction of accomplishing something on his own. In addition, the people who are trying to meet the needs of the dependent person may become tired and resentful of taking care of someone who does not even try to help himself. Further, the dependent person may miss opportunities to go places and do things because others assume they cannot or will not participate.

In my own experience, a compromise approach works best. I try to live my life as independently as possible, doing as much for myself as I physically can, while still remaining safe (Guiding Star #1), but I ask for and accept help for activities that I cannot do, or that would be dangerous to attempt on my own. For example, while my caregivers are wonderful, I also enjoy having time by myself. I need my caregivers to take me shopping and to doctors' appointments during the day, but I also enjoy my alone time in the evenings. After a recent fall, I needed to have my caregivers 24 hours per day while I recovered, but having someone with me all the time became tedious. As I became stronger, I wanted to have my alone time again, but there was concern that I was still not fully steady.

To solve the problem, I figured out a compromise. I got one of those buttons that you wear and that can summon help if you fall or otherwise need assistance, and I arranged my schedule so that I took my shower in the late afternoon when a caregiver could be there if I needed help. With those changes, my caregivers could leave at 6 pm and not return until the next morning. By accepting help (the Life Alert button and showering when my caregivers were in the apartment), I regained some independence without compromising my safety. (And after that, I gained even more independence - spending Sundays all day on my own!)

And one more thing I learned about asking for help: Don't expect people to be mind readers! Be specific and patient with them. I would often get impatient and frustrated when, after taking the hard (for me!) step of asking for help, people would ask questions about what they should do, or simply do the wrong thing. Eventually, however, I learned that I had to explain what I needed them to do. Not as much fun as mind readers, but it worked!

Guiding Star #3:
Maintain a Positive Attitude and Be Patient With Yourself. Always Treat Yourself Kindly.

The last of my three guiding stars may seem rather obvious and full of popular psychology. Yet, a positive attitude is the foundation for almost all the material in this book. If you do not at least try to have a positive attitude, there is little point in trying to make life easier or more comfortable for yourself – you won't enjoy or appreciate it anyway.

The best news, however, is that by picking up this book, you are showing a positive attitude – the hope or belief that your life with a disability can be good. That belief is the reason I wrote this book. As I stated in the Introduction, if one person's life is improved by a suggestion from this book, I will be satisfied.

But I also want readers to understand that life with a disability is not easy, and that improvement is often very slow. Life with a disability requires extraordinary patience. It requires you to be patient with others for not fully understanding your disability and what you might need, and it requires you to have extra patience and compassion for yourself, for not being able to do what you used to be able to do. Patience and compassion will go a long way toward making something that is hard, a little bit easier.

Now that I have explained my guiding stars, or rules to live by, we can get down to some of the details of how to make life easier.

Two

Home Safety and Livability

In an ideal world, after a person incurs a disability, his or her home would automatically be remodeled and redecorated to accommodate the disability. While some people do have the resources to accomplish that, most people do not. (I certainly didn't!) But there are some relatively simple modifications that can be made to make a home safer and easier for a person with a disability to live in. In this chapter, I will describe the modifications that I found helpful in my home.

Overall Floor-Plan

One-level Living

I live in a one-level condominium apartment in a high-rise building with an elevator, so navigating stairs was not an issue for me. If, however, you live in a house or apartment building that has stairs, and your disability makes it difficult for you to use those stairs, then mobility becomes hard and maybe even dangerous. Some possible solutions include:

1. Moving all the major living spaces onto one floor. A den or dining room can be made into a bedroom, but this solution can get expensive if a bathroom also has to be installed.

2. Installing a stair lift or even an elevator. These can range in expense, but compared to the next solution, they can seem downright economical.

3. Moving to a one-level home. Depending on the severity of the disability, sometimes this turns out to be the best option.

Clear Pathways

If your disability involves difficulty walking or difficulty with vision, it is helpful to have clear pathways. I made sure all the walking pathways in my home were clear and easy to navigate. I removed all the furniture that I did not need, and I also got rid of all the fragile or unsteady items, such as floor lamps, decorative tables, vases, statuaries, small rugs and knickknacks, that I might trip over or knock over.

Sturdy Furniture for Support

Since I have some difficulty with balance and weakness in my legs, I found it helpful to place sturdy furniture at intervals along the walking pathways in my home so I can reach from one to another to steady myself, similar to a toddler in the cruising stage of learning to walk.

Wheelchair Accessibility

If you will be using a wheelchair, either temporarily or permanently, it is good to have clear pathways, as described above, and it is also helpful to have as much room as possible to maneuver. In this situation, the sturdy furniture can be pushed to the sides of the rooms to maximize the traveling spaces. If doorways are too narrow, it may help to remove the doors from the hinges to provide a few extra inches. If the absence of a door causes a privacy issue, you can hang a curtain on a rod in the doorway. Bed sheets can be a great temporary curtain!

The Bathroom

Bathrooms can be dangerous places for people with physical disabilities, but there are some modifications you can make which can increase safety. The following modifications run the gamut from simple fixes to suggestions which might be helpful if you are installing a new bathroom or even building a new house.

Flooring

Tile floors are durable and can be cleaned easily, but if the tiles have a smooth surface, they can be very slippery when wet. As an alternative, I installed mold-resistant wall-to-wall carpeting, which greatly reduces the possibility of a slip and fall. For those of you who cringe at the thought of carpeting in a bathroom, a middle-ground alternative is a rough surface tile.

Shower Stall

A shower stall is generally safer than a bathtub/shower combination. A shower stall is easier to get in and out of, and does not have the curves of a tub, which can be tricky for someone with a disability. A shower stall also can accommodate a shower chair more easily than a tub, which leads to my next recommendation.

Shower Chair or Stool

Using a shower chair makes showering much safer for people who may get dizzy or have balance difficulties, or who have orthopedic problems that make standing uncomfortable. I prefer a shower chair with side arms and a back rather than a shower stool. The back and side arms make me feel more secure and less likely to topple onto the floor, but some people might find the back and side arms too restrictive, especially when using a handheld shower head (My next recommendation!).

Handheld Shower Head

I have found that using a handheld shower head makes showering easier and safer for me. Pointing the handheld shower head at various parts of my body is easier than moving my body around under the shower.

Toilet

Ideally, the toilet should be at a height that allows you to place both feet flat on the floor with your thighs parallel to the ground. Having your feet flat on the floor and your thighs parallel to the ground increases your comfort and safety, and it will also make it easier to stand up, as I will describe in the section on procedures for daily living. If the existing toilets in your home are too low, you can get an elevated toilet seat from a medical supply store or website.

Sink

As with the toilet, the bathroom sink also should be at a height that is comfortable for you, especially if you are in a wheelchair. In addition, a single lever faucet can be less complicated to operate and can reduce the possibility of scalding, compared to a dual lever faucet. Further, the vanity or counter area around the sink should be as user-friendly as possible, with ample space for soap, toothbrushes, toothpaste, etc.

Safety Bars

Safety or grab bars can make a bathroom much safer for a person with a disability. Position the bars in places where you might need to steady yourself, and make sure they are at a height where you, not the 6'4" handyman, can grab them easily. I have a 24" vertical bar installed so that I can grab it as I step into the shower, and I have another one installed directly in front of my shower chair to help me stand up.

When installing safety bars, make certain they are anchored to the wall studs and properly installed. Otherwise, they might not hold your weight when you need them. I thought my original safety bars were anchored to the studs, until one day I grabbed one and it came right out of the wall, resulting in a bad fall for me. So make sure your safety bars are properly installed!

Telephone

It never seems to fail that whenever you are in the bathroom, the telephone will ring. With the advent of answering machines and voicemail, many people are able to withstand the urge to run to answer the phone, but there may be that one important call that you have been waiting for and do not want to miss. When you are young and physically able, running for the phone is not a big deal, but when a physical disability is involved, running for the phone, especially from the bathroom, can be a recipe for disaster. Therefore, it can be a good idea to have a cordless phone in your bathroom. It could also be a lifesaver in the event of a medical emergency.

The Kitchen

Many accidents occur in the kitchen. People often are more fearful of falls in the bathroom, which can cause broken bones or head injuries, but kitchen accidents, such as a kitchen fire, can also be quite dangerous. Kitchen accidents involving broken glass or spilled liquids can result in serious cuts or falls, and even if no injuries result, kitchen accidents involving spills or breakage can be just plain messy and frustrating. Therefore, in this section, I recommend ways in which your kitchen can become safer and more user-friendly for a person with a disability.

Clear Counters and Work Areas

Make your counters and work areas as clutter-free as possible. Fewer items on a counter mean fewer things that can be knocked over or off the counter.

Microwave Oven

I feel more comfortable using a microwave oven instead of the stove or the standard oven. Although a microwave can heat foods to the point where they can cause burns, the oven itself does not get hot (unlike a stove or conventional oven). In addition, the microwave will shut off when the cooking time is up – I do not have to worry about forgetting to turn it off. Therefore, I highly recommend having a microwave in your kitchen.

Organized Refrigerator and Freezer

Since I am blind, it is extremely helpful for me to have my refrigerator and freezer very organized. I designate certain shelves or areas for specific food items, so I don't have to search for them. I also try to limit the number of food items in my refrigerator and freezer so they do not get too crowded. A less crowded space makes it easier to find what you are looking for, and it lessens the chance of items tumbling out or spilling during your search. (This can also be helpful for someone with movement or balance difficulties.) Another hint for the refrigerator is to try to avoid glass bottles or containers, so that if something does tumble out, you do not have broken glass to clean up. A final hint for the refrigerator and freezer is to label food storage containers with the food name and date of storage. I use raised stick-on numbers and letters that can be purchased for labeling. The labels help me to determine what is safe to be eaten, and what should be thrown out, which also help to de-clutter my refrigerator and freezer.

Dishes and Glassware

I like plastic or other non-breakable dishes and tableware, so I don't have to worry about getting cut after dropping a dish. I make certain they are safe for both the dishwasher and the microwave.

Dishwasher

If you are visually-challenged or have limited movement, it may be best to wash dishes by hand, or have someone else load and unload the dishwasher. It can be time-consuming and frustrating for someone who is visually-impaired to try to put the dishes into the racks, and the repetitive bending and reaching involved in loading and unloading a dishwasher can be tiring or even dangerous for someone with limited movement. Also, whether you use the dishwasher, or wash dishes by hand and put them in a dish rack to dry, it is safer to place the knives with the blade pointing down, to avoid getting cut or stabbed as you reach over the utensils.

The Bedroom

For the bedroom, my main recommendation is to repeat what I said earlier about having clear pathways. Try to keep pillows, comforters and bedspreads off the floor, especially on the path to the bathroom, so you do not trip over them in the middle of the night. Some other suggestions are as follows:

Telephone

It can be helpful to have a telephone on a nightstand next to your bed so you do not have to get out of bed to answer the phone in the middle of the night. It also might be a lifesaver if you have to call for help in the event of a medical emergency.

Alerting Device

At one point during my medical odyssey of various ailments and injuries, I was too weak to get out of bed without assistance, but I kept forgetting that fact, and I would try to get out of bed by myself to go to the bathroom, and would often end up on the floor. Fortunately, a visiting nurse or therapist (I cannot remember exactly who it was) recommended a device by Medline called the Advantage Magnetic Alarm. A magnetic sensor attaches to the patient and also to a cord leading to the alarm. If the patient tries to get out of bed without assistance, the sensor will dislodge and the alarm will sound. This device also might be useful for someone who sleepwalks, or for someone who wakes up groggy and might need a few minutes to collect themselves before getting out of bed.

An Organized Clothes Closet

A well-organized clothes closet can save time and avoid needless frustration. Try not to have items stacked up high that can tumble down onto your head. Since I am blind and have difficulty coordinating outfits, a friend of mine arranges my clothing into outfits (slacks or skirts with matching tops) that are either hung on one hanger or on multiple hangers held together with a Scrunci (the fabric covered hair tie which works better for this purpose than a rubber band).

Clothing

And now a word or two about clothing: To remain as independent as possible, it is helpful to have clothing that allows you to dress yourself. If buttoning a button is difficult for you, buy clothes that fasten with snaps or Velcro, or have the buttons on your existing clothing replaced with snaps or Velcro.

Another clothing tip is to buy clothing with pockets so that certain items such as eyeglasses, facial tissues, an inhaler, and especially a cell phone or cordless phone, can be with you at all times. If mobility is difficult for you, it can be annoying, tiring, and even life-threatening, to have to cross a room or walk to another room to retrieve one of those items. If you are having trouble finding clothes you like that have usable pockets (it seems to me that manufacturers are not putting pockets on clothing as much as they used to!), or if you have some favorite outfits that do not have usable pockets, a solution I have used is to buy some coordinating fabric at a fabric store and have pockets put on the clothes that need them.

A final clothing suggestion is to wear clothing that is comfortable for you. A disability usually comes with enough health and pain issues, so you do not want to add to them by wearing clothing that causes skin irritations, rashes, or sores.

Three

Mobility and Self-Care

In the previous chapter, I suggested some ways to make your home (and your clothing) easier and safer for you to live in. In this chapter, I will describe some procedures and suggestions that can help with the activities of your daily living.

Getting out of Bed

If it is physically difficult for you to get out of bed, a simple maneuver called the "log-rolling technique" may make it easier for you. The log-rolling technique involves the following steps:

STEP 1:   Lie on your back, and then slowly move your body so that you are lying close to one side of the bed. About five to six inches from the edge is best – any closer and you might accidentally log roll yourself right off the bed!

STEP 2:   Roll onto your side, facing the edge of the bed and keeping your back straight.

STEP 3:   Bend your knees so that your knees and lower legs extend beyond the edge of the bed.

STEP 4:   Take a deep breath and let your feet slowly fall to the floor. The weight of your feet falling to the floor will raise your upper body to a sitting position, so that you are sitting on the side of the bed with both feet on the floor. You can use your elbow to help push yourself up and your hands to help steady you.

STEP 5:   Once you are in a seated position, take a few deep breaths to make sure there is enough oxygen in your brain before you attempt to stand up.

Standing up from a Seated Position

Whether sitting on the edge of the bed, or on the toilet, or on a sofa, chair or park bench, getting up from a seated position can be challenging for those with certain physical disabilities or the infirmities that come with a ripe old age. Recently, my daughter was at a shopping center when an elderly woman seated on a bench asked for her help in getting up. The woman said she had been trying unsuccessfully to get up for nearly half an hour. The following simple method, taught to me by my third or fourth physical therapist, probably would have helped that woman get up by herself. I know it has helped me get up from a seated position on my own, and has thereby helped me to maintain more of my independence in my everyday life.

STEP 1: Place your feet flat on the ground in front of you – shoulder-width apart – with your lower legs perpendicular to the floor.

STEP 2: Bend forward from your hips until your nose is directly above an imaginary line running from the toes of one foot to the toes of the other.

STEP 3: Stretch your arm out in front of you to help balance yourself, and try standing up. You will be amazed at how much easier it is.

Walking Independently

Once you are standing up, the next step (pardon the pun!) is walking. Since I became blind, I am much less sure of my balance when I am walking. A physical therapist taught me a way of standing and walking that helps me to feel more secure. It is not pretty, and it is the antithesis of the "walk" taught to beauty pageant contestants, but it helps me to get around safely so I am willing to use it.

STEP 1: Bend your arms at the elbows and move them a few inches away from your body.

STEP 2: Keep your feet shoulder-width apart and your knees slightly bent.

STEP 3: To increase your sense of balance, raise one arm so that your hand is approximately one foot in front of your face with the palm turn outward, as though you are shielding your face.

STEP 4: Try to keep your chin parallel with the floor.

Although this way of walking may lack sex appeal, it gets me where I am going safely, which is better than ending up on the floor.

Walking with the Assistance of a Walker or Cane

The main point of the previous section is to get where you are going safely, and that theme continues in this section. It is bad for your health, both mentally and physically, to sit and do nothing all day. A person with a disability or the infirmities of old age needs to keep the rest of his or her body moving, in order to avoid additional complications. That being said, however, the goal is to move safely. Falls can be messy and embarrassing, and can cause serious injuries that can lead to additional disabilities. Therefore, there is no shame in using a walker or cane to help you get where you are going safely.

I am going to repeat that last sentence. **There is no embarrassment or shame in using a walker or cane!** I am always amazed at how many people refuse to use a walker or cane due to pride or fear of embarrassment. In my view, the only shame is when people refuse to use a walker, and end up falling and causing themselves additional injury and disability, or staying home and depriving themselves of opportunities to socialize with family and friends.

I use a walker that has wheels, a seat, and a basket. I like the feeling of stability it gives me, and the seat is useful when I have to wait somewhere or when I get tired and need a break. In addition, the basket is useful for carrying my purse when I am shopping.

I also use a cane from time to time, specifically a quad cane because it is more stable. It does not provide quite as much stability as my walker, but it is more portable and easier to maneuver in tight quarters.

Whether you use a walker or a cane, it is important to have a physical therapist fit it to your unique body. A hand-me-down cane or walker may be financially appealing, but if it causes your back to ache or does not provide adequate stability, it may be doing more harm than good.

Similarly, the physical therapist should teach you the correct way to use the walker or cane, in order to prevent accidents or injuries. Although using a cane or walker may seem pretty basic and self-explanatory, you would be surprised at how many people suffer preventable injuries from improper use. For example, a walker should not be used to pull oneself up to a standing position, especially if it has wheels. If something is movable or light enough for you to pick up easily, it is not safe to support your weight!

Walking with the Assistance of a Person

While remaining as independent as possible is one of my main goals, there are times when, due to my blindness, I need someone to assist me when I walk. After much trial and error, my caregivers and I have come up with the following system of walking together that works well for us.

When walking with one of my caregivers, I stand very close but one-half step behind her, with my hand through the crook of her bent arm. In this way, she is leading me, not pushing or pulling me. I find that being led is very similar to dancing with a partner – one leads while the other follows. For me, being led is much preferable to being pushed or pulled, which I find very disconcerting due to my blindness.

My caregiver warns me in advance of steps, curbs, low branches, furniture, etc., and if an impediment is suddenly directly in front of me, she uses the word "Stop" to alert me. Upon hearing the word, "Stop," I halt immediately, and then my caregiver tells me what the impediment is and how we can get around it. We have found that the one-word "Stop" system works better than phrases such as "Watch your step" or "There is something in your way," which can be confusing and can waste the precious time between when the caregiver notices the impediment and I end up tripping over it.

I live in Florida where it is warm and humid for much of the year, and people tend to get sweaty. My caregivers and I have found that putting my sweaty hand into the crook of their sweaty arms was kind of yucky. To solve that problem, I wear short white cotton gloves on my hands whenever we are walking together. The gloves are inexpensive, machine washable, do not shrink, and come in several sizes. We found them at Walgreen's, but they are probably available at other drugstores or discount stores too.

One final tip about walking, whether unassisted or with a cane, walker, or another person: Wears safe shoes! Shoes that have higher heels, platforms or smooth soles can make a fall more likely. Even if you have worn such shoes your whole life, they can become more dangerous when your mobility is impaired by a disability or increasing age. Therefore, to increase your safety, wear flat, supportive shoes with a non-skid sole. They may not be as attractive as the shoes you used to wear, but they are definitely more attractive than a broken hip!

Brushing Teeth

If you have loss of vision or trembling hands, putting toothpaste on a toothbrush can seem like an impossible task. The following procedure can make tooth brushing easy again, and help you maintain your dental health (so you do not add mouth problems to your list of disabilities!):

STEP 1:   Squeeze a dab of toothpaste onto your tongue.

STEP 2:   Wet the toothbrush.

STEP 3:   Place the toothbrush on the dab of toothpaste and proceed to brush your teeth.

Drying Off After a Shower or Bath, and Getting Dressed

When balance, stability and/or movement are a problem for you, drying yourself off after a shower or bath, and getting dressed, can become challenging, if not downright dangerous. To make it easier and safer, my caregivers and I have developed the following procedure:

STEP 1:   Before getting into the shower or bath, spread a towel out near the edge of the bed (where you are able to sit) and hang another large bath towel next to the shower or bath. Next to the towel on the bed, set out the clothing you will be putting on, as well as any creams or deodorants you plan to use. If you are not showering or bathing at this time, but are just getting dressed, skip to Step 4.

STEP 2:   When you exit the shower or bath, take several breaths to make sure your head is clear and you are not dizzy (You may want to hold onto a safety bar, if you have one). Then wrap the large towel around you, and wipe your feet dry on the bath mat.

STEP 3:   Walk to the bed, sit down on the towel that has been spread out, and then dry off completely. It is much safer to dry yourself off from a seated position. You are less likely to lose your balance and topple over as you reach to dry your legs or other out-of-the-way places.

STEP 4: Put on any deodorants, creams, or ointments. As described above, it is much easier and safer to do this from a seated position.

STEP 5: Put on your clothing. Again, it is much safer to do this from a seated position. Before becoming disabled, you may have been able to step into your pants or skirt while standing (maybe even both legs at once!), but since disabilities often affect balance and stability, it is much safer, and therefore smarter, to put on your clothing while sitting down.

Four

Vision Loss

As you have probably noticed, many of the suggestions in this book come from the point of view of someone with vision loss, because that is one of my disabilities, but they also are applicable to people with a variety of disabilities. The following suggestions, however, are geared specifically to those individuals with some loss of vision:

Adaptive Devices and Equipment

Explore the many adaptive devices and equipment developed for people with vision loss, and find out what is helpful to you. Some examples of adaptive devices and equipment are talking clocks, talking watches, large-button telephones, and pens with darker ink. Resources to help you find out about such items include catalogs, websites, and agencies that provide services for people with vision loss.

Maximize Light

Have as much light as you can in your home. Even though you may have lost much of your vision, increased light can help you make the most of what remains, which can increase your feelings of safety and security. This is especially true at night. It can be helpful to leave some lights on when you go to sleep at night, so that you will not have to fumble to find the light switch if you should need to get up in the middle of the night.

Five

Hearing Loss

I also have significant hearing loss, so here are some suggestions that I have found helpful.

Hearing Aids

Get the best hearing aids you can afford, and wear them! Some people resist wearing hearing aids because they think it will make them look old or "out of it." Believe me, the people who really look old or out of touch are those who are constantly saying "What?! What did you say?" and those who cannot hear enough to partake in the conversation. If you do not believe me, ask any younger person who interacts with a person with hearing loss!

Adaptive Devices and Equipment

As with vision loss, find out about all the adaptive devices and equipment that are available to aid those with hearing loss. Some that I have found helpful are amplified telephones and smoke detectors, and attachments that amplify the doorbell. As noted above with respect to vision loss, resources include catalogs, websites and agencies that serve those with hearing loss.

Location, Location, Location!

Try to position yourself and modify your surroundings (to the extent possible depending on the situation) so as to maximize your ability to hear. Try to avoid noisy settings, such as noisy restaurants. Within various settings, try to find the quietest areas. In restaurants, the quietest areas tend to be away from the entry and the kitchen. Quieter settings tend to have more carpet, upholstery, and draperies, instead of hard surfaces, such as wood or concrete floors.

Eliminate Background Noise

Try to eliminate background noise as much as possible. In your own home, turn off the radio or television when you are trying to have a conversation.

Let People Know How to Communicate with You

You can tell the people you frequently interact with about the following suggestions for communicating with a person with hearing loss:

Suggestion 1: Move closer to the person with hearing loss before you begin speaking. The ideal distance is to be within three to six feet.

Suggestion 2: Face the person with hearing loss before you begin to speak, and talk directly to him or her. By facing the person, you provide valuable extra information such as the position of your lips, and your facial, hand and body gestures, which can fill in for the sounds they might not be able to hear. Try not to turn away while you are speaking, because that will significantly reduce the volume of your speech.

Suggestion 3: Refrain from eating, drinking, or chewing gum while speaking, because those activities will garble what you are saying.

Suggestion 4: Introduce a topic clearly, rather than launching right in. For example, "Dad (pause), I want to talk about your trip to Florida," rather than, "What time is your flight?" If you are discussing a complicated topic, some good organization and clear transitions will aid understanding.

Suggestion 5: In group conversations, try to have only one person speak at a time, and if possible, the person about to speak should provide a subtle visual cue, such as a hand gesture, so that the person with hearing loss can turn to face that person.

Six

Obtaining Health Care

Having a disability or the infirmities of advanced age often means frequent contact with doctors, hospitals and other health care providers. While most of us would like to believe that all health care providers put their patients' best interests above financial or personal concerns, that belief may be naïve. Instead of practicing independently, many doctors are now employed by large healthcare systems that pressure them to produce revenue and meet practice guidelines. Similarly, most hospitals are now run as businesses, whether they are considered "non-profit" or "for profit." Accordingly, you cannot dependably rely on health care providers to put your best interests before cost and convenience.

Also, health care has become more complicated, with multiple doctors often involved in providing treatment, so miscommunications or failures to communicate can occur. In addition, the pressure to cut costs means that many health care providers are overworked and stretched too thin, and many health care institutions are staffed with employees who have less education and experience than you might think. In short, there are lots of ways in which your health care could go wrong, or not as well as it could have gone. Therefore, in this chapter, I give some suggestions for increasing your chances of obtaining the best possible health care and health care outcomes.

Be Informed

Get as much information as you can before you make a decision. Some of the areas in which you should obtain information are as follows:

Doctors

Choose your doctors carefully. Ask for recommendations from family, friends, and especially other health care providers and workers, and ask why they chose that doctor. You can also obtain information about doctors, including where they were educated and any malpractice claims, from medical agencies or Internet websites. Finally, if after meeting with a doctor, you do not feel comfortable with him or her, consider switching to another doctor. Notice that I said "consider." Before making a change, remember that the main goal is to get the best medical treatment for your ailment. I would choose medical expertise over a good bedside manner in almost every situation.

Treatments

Find out as much as you can about your diagnosis. The Internet may be one of the first places you look for information, and there is plenty of information there, but remember that not all of it is accurate and comes from legitimate sources. Websites of foundations or support groups for your disease or ailment, such as The Leukemia and Lymphoma Society, can be a good resource – they usually will have a list of resources or have their own books and pamphlets. If you have any doubts or uncertainty about whether the diagnosis is accurate, get a second opinion from another doctor. In addition, ask your friends, neighbors, co-workers, etc. if they know anything about your disease or ailment, or know anyone else who does. Although you always have to consider the sources and take everything with a grain of salt, friends and acquaintances can provide tips on good health care providers, where to get medical supplies, or how to manage possible side effects of treatment, etc. I realize some people may prefer to be more private about their disease or ailment, and I am not advocating sharing more information than you feel comfortable disclosing, but you never know when a friend of a friend might provide you with useful (or even life-saving) information.

Medications

Find out as much as you can about all the medications you take. Read the information that comes with the drug, talk to your pharmacist, and ask your doctor what other patients have experienced while taking that drug. You can also look on the Internet (again, remember to consider the source of Internet information). Find out about side effects and drug interactions, and also how various foods might affect how it works. The more you know about your medications, the less likely you will be to experience unpleasant drug interactions, or side effects that could easily have been avoided with some advance planning (such as eating lots of fiber or taking a mild laxative if one of your medications tends to cause constipation).

Keep a Medical Log and Medication Chart

Once you have found out information about the various drugs you are taking, it is helpful to organize it into a chart, so you and your health care providers can see how it all fits together. The chart can list each medication, the dosage, when you take it, when you began taking it, drug interactions, food interactions, and side effects. You can bring the chart with you to all your doctor appointments, so your doctor can avoid prescribing a drug that might interfere with the effectiveness of another drug you are already taking.

In addition, to a medication chart, it is also helpful to have a medical log to keep track of all your doctors' appointments and medical procedures. With many disabilities and with the infirmities that come with advanced age, it can seem as though you are constantly visiting doctors or having medical tests or procedures. To keep track of when I last saw a certain doctor or had a specific test, I use a medical log, which is just a notebook in which I write down the date, the name of the health care provider I saw, the reason for the visit, and any procedures or tests that were done. I bring it to every medical appointment, so I do not have to struggle to remember when I last saw the dentist or had a chest X-ray. My medical log is in the low-tech form of a pen and notebook, but if you are technically savvy, or have a friend or relative who is, your medical log (and your medication chart) could be in the form of a computer file or database. (Just make sure you back up the file and make a hard copy from time to time!)

Have a Health Care Buddy

It can be very stressful to be a patient, especially in today's fast-paced health care environment. Doctors, nurses, and other health care workers often provide information at the same time they are doing an exam or procedure, so a patient who is dutifully trying to follow the doctor's direction to "Take a deep breath and hold it" may not always hear everything the doctor is saying about their condition. That is especially true when the patient has just heard or is afraid of hearing bad news about his or her health. Therefore, I recommend having a "health care buddy" accompany you to doctors' appointments and other medical situations.

The health care buddy can serve as your extra brain – listening and remembering what the doctor says, and asking questions you might not think of until after the doctor has left. The health care buddy can be a spouse, sibling, adult child, or a friend. It is helpful if you can have the same person be your health care buddy for most, if not all, of your doctor and medical appointments. By having just one person, rather than various people, that one person can become familiar with your medical conditions, will better understand what the doctor is saying, and will have some idea of what questions to ask. Of course not everyone has someone who can be so available and is willing to come to every appointment. In that case, several health care buddies are better than none.

Be Extra Careful During Hospital Stays

The hospital is one place where it is very helpful to have a health care buddy with you. Many people have the feeling that once they check into the hospital, they can relax - their physical well-being is now in the hands of the experts. In some ways that is true; their vital signs and the symptoms of their illness are constantly being monitored, and treatment decisions will be made and implemented by licensed medical personnel. In other ways, however, a hospital stay is a situation requiring extra vigilance. As noted earlier, many hospitals are understaffed, and the staff they do have may be inexperienced and overworked. When you have lots of sick people, with all different kinds of ailments, all together in one place, it is not uncommon for mistakes to be made and diseases transmitted.

Most likely, if you are hospitalized, you are not your most alert and vigilant self. A health care buddy can be your eyes, ears and brain, while you are working on resting and getting your body well. Your health care buddy can listen to what the doctors and other professionals say about your condition, can watch what the various professionals do as they attend to you in your hospital room, and can put two and two together to try to make sure you are getting the care you need – for example, asking "Didn't the doctor say that she should be helped to walk in the hallway at least twice per day?" or "The nurse on the morning shift said that someone on the afternoon shift would be in to change the bandage. Will you be doing that?" Of course, your health care buddy should not be obnoxious or demanding – that would do more harm than good – but simply observing and asking some simple questions if something seems to have been forgotten or contrary to the doctor's directions can help to keep your hospital care on track.

If your health care buddy cannot be there at all times (you shouldn't be offended – most people cannot, because of work or family obligations, or their own health concerns, such as needing to get some sleep so they don't get sick!), you might ask other family members or friends to stand in, or even consider hiring a private caregiver or nurse. Although private care can be expensive, it may be worth it, depending on your medical condition and how able you are to monitor your own care.

Another way to be extra careful during hospital stays is to bring copies of your medical log and your medication chart. The medical log and medication chart can help if questions come up about whether you have had a certain test or tried a specific medication, and can also help to avoid unfortunate drug interactions.

Also, during hospital stays, it is best to leave all your valuables at home. A hospital stay is not the time to be worrying about the safety of your jewelry, or mourning the loss or theft of your jewelry. Lock it up and leave it at home or with a friend.

In addition, to make your hospital stay as stress free as possible, try to arrange for any special requests in advance. If you would like a private room, you can request that, but also be sure to ask about any additional cost. Once you are in your room, if there is something that is hindering your ability to rest and get well, such as a roommate who snores like a chainsaw all night, ask if a change can be made. Also, be sure to ask for any special equipment, such as a commode chair, that you are using at home or that might be helpful to you during your hospital stay. If you are using a commode chair at home, you probably also should be using one at the hospital. There is no reason to fall and break your hip on the way to the bathroom, just because you are in the hospital and not at home.

Speaking of falling and breaking your hip, please watch your step in the hospital room! Hospital rooms can be rather dangerous places, especially for the disabled and/or infirm. The floors are often slippery, and there can be obstacles to trip over, such as IV stands and movable bedside tables. In addition, the hospital room is usually an unfamiliar place, and can be disorienting to someone waking up in the middle of the night, groggy from medication. Therefore, before you get up in the middle of the night to go to the bathroom, sit on the edge of the bed for a minute to get your bearings and adjust your vision to the low light, and then step carefully on your way to the bathroom. And if you need assistance, by all means ask for it!

A hospital stay is not the time to demonstrate how independent (stubborn? foolish?) you are, and as I have noted before, there is no need to fall and break a hip, and thereby add to your disabilities.

Plan as Much as You Can for Post-Hospital Care, or at Least Be Aware of Some Options.

If you are having a planned surgery, such as a hip replacement, which will cause you to need some assistance afterward, you can find out from the doctor what type of limitations you might have following the surgery. Then you, or your spouse or other family member, can make appropriate arrangements for your care. That is the easy scenario. Your needs are known in advance and generally of limited duration. Family and friends can plan in advance to help out for a short period of time.

Unfortunately, there is often another scenario – the hard one. We usually do not know when life is going to blindside us. One day we are fully functional and self-sufficient, and then the next day we might be in the hospital, struggling with the effects of a serious stroke, fall or accident, or in my case, a serious and sudden illness.

Most people who are hospitalized just want to go home, but satisfying that desire is not always easy. Hospital stays are generally limited to acute care, so patients often are discharged to a rehabilitation facility to continue their recovery. How soon they are able to return to their homes often depends on who is available to take care of them at home. The potential caregivers might include a spouse, children, grandchildren, friends, neighbors, paid caregivers, or some combination these people, and an important consideration is whether the caregiver(s) you choose (or that are chosen for you) will be able to provide you with the care you need.

My recommendation is to think through these issues ahead of time. What arrangements would you like to have if you have a serious illness or disability that causes you to be less than self-sufficient for more than a few weeks? In the next chapter, I discuss in-home care and what I have learned about making it work as well as possible.

Seven

In-Home Care

The need for in-home care can be sudden. In my situation, a serious illness took away my eyesight in a matter of days, and took my independence along with it. It also can occur gradually, such as when disease or the infirmities of old age advance to the point where the person can no longer be self-sufficient. Most people do not like to think about needing care, so they often are unprepared when the need arises. As a result, the person, or more likely his or her family, must scramble to meet an existing need.

Gather Information before the Need Arises

As noted in the previous chapter, potential caregivers include the spouse, children, grandchildren, siblings, other relatives, friends, neighbors, and paid caregivers. The spouse usually just assumes the role of primary caregiver, and that arrangement works fine....until it doesn't. The spouse might become ill, or even die, or just may not be capable of providing all the care that is needed, either because of physical limitations (unable to lift or support the patient in getting out of bed or using the bathroom) or inability to handle medical needs such as changing dressings, administering medications, or monitoring medical conditions, or just plain exhaustion. At that point, or initially if there is no spouse, decisions must be made. Can family members provide all the care and assistance that is needed, or is paid help necessary? Is there enough money to provide for in-home care, or must the person move to an assisted living facility or nursing home to provide the level of care that is needed?

If you are the person who needs care, you will probably want to have as much input into these decisions as possible. Therefore, it is wise to gather as much information as possible about care options in your area so that you know what care options you would like if the need should arise. Otherwise, you might find yourself in a situation you do not like because you had no alternative to suggest when the need arose.

In exploring your options and making your plans, it may be helpful to talk to a geriatric or home health care social worker who can tell you what options (for home health or rehabilitative care) are available in your area. In addition to paid caregivers and agencies, there may be non-profit agencies that provide services, such as Meals on Wheels, adult day care, volunteer visits, or rides to doctor's appointments. Such services may help to fill in gaps in care provided by other caregivers. Also, talk to friends or neighbors who may have already faced these issues. If they hired caregivers, ask for the name of the agency, if they went through an agency, and ask for the names of any caregivers they especially liked. (Be extra careful about hiring caregivers not with an agency. Check references carefully! There are too many instances of caregivers turning out to be thieves or worse.)

And a special caveat for people who are planning to rely on family members and compensate them financially by transferring assets to them: Consult with an experienced attorney before you make any arrangements! Sometimes the arrangements can backfire. For example, an elderly woman might offer to have her son and his family come to live with her and take care of her as she ages, in exchange for putting his name on the deed to her house so that he will inherit it when she dies. Such an arrangement might work well in some cases, but what if they do not all get along, and the son and his family decide to move out. The woman might then decide to sell her house and move into an assisted living facility, but since her son is now a co-owner, she might have to buy him out before she can sell. What a mess!

So, my advice is to do your research to find out what is available in your area, but do not make any permanent arrangements involving money or other assets without consulting a knowledgeable attorney or financial planner.

If the Care Arrangement Is Not Working, Change It

Another piece of advice is not to be afraid to change your arrangements if you are not happy with them. The following story of my experience with paid caregivers is a good lesson in how even the best-laid plans do not always work out as you expect.

My Experience with In-Home Care

A year or so before my temporal arteritis struck, when I was still fully independent and merrily living my life, I became friendly with a neighbor who operated a care-giving agency. Several other neighbors in our condominium building were using her services, and she seemed very nice and reliable. Since one of my former jobs involved overseeing home health care services, I was aware that many people eventually need care of some type. And because I was, and still am, determined to remain in my own home, and since I have no family in the area, I knew that I was a likely candidate to need some type of in-home care at some point. Accordingly, I talked with this woman (I'll call her Kay for purposes of this book), about providing care for me if I would ever need it.

Thus, when my ophthalmologist told me I needed to go directly to the hospital for treatment to try to save my eyesight, I called Kay to accompany me and be my "hospital buddy." (I have a very close friend whom I'll call Mary, and whom I have named as my "Health Care Surrogate," but she was not available that day.) At that time, I felt fortunate that there was someone I could call, and then when I lost my eyesight two days later, I felt that I had been quite prudent and foresighted. Kay and her care-giving employees stayed with me in the hospital during that traumatic time, and were available to provide 24-hour care in my home upon my discharge from the hospital. Because of that, I did not have to go to a rehabilitation hospital or nursing home. It seemed that my advance planning was working out quite well!

Unfortunately (and here is an important lesson!), the best-laid plans do not always turn out as we expect. Once I was at home, and quite depressed and vulnerable due to my sudden blindness, Kay became very domineering and controlling. She began a complete clean-out of my apartment, encouraging me to give away many of my treasured possessions because "you won't need that anymore since you are blind," or to eliminate everything that might be potential hazards. I still do not know what happened to some of my things. She also tried to baby me and keep me dependent on her, discouraging my attempts to do things for myself. In addition, she encouraged my over-medication, giving me sleeping pills and other medicines that made me feel groggy much of the time.

Luckily, I had given my daughter a power of attorney to handle my finances. Otherwise, Kay may have invaded that part of my life, with terrible consequences for my financial well-being. Kay did, however, try to manipulate my daughter and my friend Mary into believing that I was being difficult every time I tried to assert some independence.

The situation grew worse and worse, but I was getting stronger and more certain that Kay and her employees were mainly looking out for themselves, and were not helping me to live the life I wanted to lead. Finally, at the recommendation of a homecare social worker, I fired Kay and her agency, and began using another agency that suited my needs much better. The new agency did not assume responsibility for my care. Instead, it referred independent contractor care-givers whom I paid directly. This type of arrangement worked well for me. I went through many caregivers during my first year with that agency, because many of the caregivers did not meet my needs – I am blind, but not senile, and I want to live an active life. I do not need a babysitter!

Eventually, I found some wonderful caregivers who have helped to make my life very full and enjoyable. Finding those caregivers took much trial and error (and a not inconsequential amount of emotional stress to the caregivers, the agency and me). In order to reduce the stress you might experience, I want to share with you what I have learned about finding the right caregivers.

First, prioritize your needs. No one is a jack-of-all-trades, so be clear about what you want your caregiver to be able to do. Does he or she need to be able to drive? Lift you in or out of bed? Be a health care buddy at doctor's appointments? Cook delicious meals? Figure out what is important to you so that you do not become frustrated with caregivers who clearly are not suited for your needs.

Second, look for personal compatibility. You will be spending a lot of time with this person, so it is best if you enjoy being with him or her. If someone is too negative for you, complaining about their troubles all day and leaving you feeling depressed, that person is not the right caregiver for you. Or if your caregiver is too hyper and perky, making you feel anxious or on edge, that person may not be a good fit for you. In other words, if for whatever reason, you breathe a sigh of relief when your caregiver walks out the door at the end of the day, it is probably best to look for a different caregiver.

I truly enjoy the company of my caregivers. We have similar senses of humor, so we laugh frequently throughout the day, and laughter is wonderful medicine!

Third, communicate with your caregivers. Most people are not mind readers. If something is important to you that they are doing or not doing, let them know.

In summary, determining the care arrangements you need and want, and finding people to provide that care, is not easy. My advice is to 1) collect information and consider the possibilities before the need arises, 2) make the best decision you can at the time the need arises, 3) try your best to make the arrangement work, and 4) do not be afraid to make changes if the arrangement is not working.

Finding the right care arrangement is a major action you can take to make it easier to live with your disability. Considering such big-picture decisions can be important to your well-being, but it can also be helpful to look at smaller fixes that may add significantly to your quality of life. In the next chapter, I describe some health or physical problems that can be prevented or remedied relatively easily, and thus avoid or alleviate pain and distress.

Eight

More Health Care Advice

Since I have been on the receiving end of quite a bit of health care during the past four years (and I worked in the health care field for many years before that), I have a few other health care-related tips that I would like to share.

Having Blood Drawn

Physicians routinely request blood tests to screen for a variety of ailments. Some people have no problem having their blood drawn. For them, a blood draw is a simple procedure requiring only a quick pinch; the worst part might be the time spent in the waiting room. For other people, however, blood draws can be difficult and painful, requiring multiple "sticks" to find a suitable vein. If you are among the latter group, there are ways to make the experience less painful.

First, check with the lab to find out if you have to refrain from eating or drinking before the test. Even if it is a fasting blood test, however, you should still be allowed to drink water. Drinking water will prevent you from becoming dehydrated and will also increase your blood volume (the amount of blood) which will make your blood easier to draw.

Second, inform the phlebotomist (the person performing the blood draw) that you have had difficulty with blood draws in the past. The phlebotomist may ask a more skilled or experienced phlebotomist, if one is available, to do your blood draw. You can also request that the phlebotomist use a butterfly needle. A butterfly needle is smaller, and may be less painful when it is inserted into your vein, but it may also cause the blood draw to take longer to complete.

After a blood draw, some people develop a large black and blue mark at the site of the needle stick. One way to try to avoid that black and blue mark is to raise your arm after the blood draw (the arm the blood came from!) above your head few minutes and apply pressure on the site of the needle stick.

Common Physical Ailments

When one part of a person's body becomes disabled, other parts of the body may be affected for various reasons, such as increased time in bed, lack of exercise, etc. Some of these effects may be painful or reduce a person's quality of life, but often they can be prevented or remedied rather easily. In this chapter, I discuss several common health problems and some relatively easy fixes. The fixes may not work in every case, but they are worth a try.

Foot Drop

Foot Drop occurs when the muscles in the foot become so weak that the person is not able to lift the front part of the foot in order to walk. One common cause of foot drop is not keeping the foot in proper alignment, which can occur if a person is confined to a bed or wheelchair for a long period of time without any support for his feet. The foot muscles relax and lose their tone, and then when the person is finally well enough to try to walk, the feet will flap instead of stepping.

To prevent foot drop, I suggest using pillows to prop up the feet so that they remain straight. When a person is lying in bed, the feet should be perpendicular to the bed, pointing toward the ceiling. A pillow can also be place under the calf to relieve pressure on the heel and prevent bed sores from developing. In a wheelchair, a pillow can be positioned against each padded footboard to keep each foot from flopping to the side. The feet should also be massaged regularly, at least once or twice per day, and the person should be encouraged to exercise the feet as much as possible.

Back Pain

I have had a bad back for many years. I have tried different types of mattresses and beds, but what has relieved my pain the most is a memory foam mattress topper. It is less expensive than a new mattress and comes in various sizes and thicknesses.

Incontinence

There are many causes of incontinence, and it can be temporary or long-term. The first step in dealing with incontinence is to talk to your doctor. Although it can be an embarrassing subject to broach, your doctor may be able to offer some ways to reduce or even solve the problem. Some possible courses of action may include medication (or changing or reducing certain medications), physical therapy, or even surgery.

If, after talking with your doctor, you determine that simply living with your incontinence is your preferred, or only, option, there are products that can make living with incontinence easier. Bed pads, either washable or disposable, can reduce the need to wash your sheets every day. The washable bed pads are more economical since they can be reused, but they do involve more work (washing them!). The disposable bed pads, which are used in hospitals, are more convenient but also more costly for long-term use. Both types are usually available at drugstores or retailers such as Wal-Mart or Target. Speaking of cost, it is probably also a good idea to invest in a rubber-backed mattress cover to protect your mattress. A rubber-backed mattress cover is much cheaper than buying a new mattress!

Irregularity

A physical disability often results in less movement and exercise, and one of the side effects of less movement and exercise may be irregularity. One approach to irregularity is to get moving again. Ask your doctor or physical therapist which exercises you can do with your disability. Sometimes, however, periods of inactivity are unavoidable (stroke, broken bones, illness, etc.), and irregularity becomes a problem. This can be especially true following surgery, when anesthesia and prolonged bed-rest can be a recipe for constipation. While some people find laxatives to be helpful and effective, particularly for acute situations such as post-surgery), I have found that adding apples and prunes to my diet has enabled me to maintain my regularity over the long-term without the harsh side-effects of laxatives. I add pitted prunes or cut-up apples to my cereal in the morning or eat them as snacks, and thereby get the fiber I need to keep things moving in the right direction.

Indigestion

As you get older, indigestion may become a more frequent problem. Foods that you used to eat with impunity may now bite you back, punishing you with heartburn or acid reflux. In addition to, or possibly even instead of, all the prescription and non-prescription medications promoted to prevent or treat indigestion, I recommend a simple technique to avoid indigestion – eat slowly, chewing your food thoroughly. Digestion begins in the mouth, and the more time the food spends in the mouth, mixing with saliva and breaking down into smaller pieces, the less time it has to spend in the stomach where all the trouble can start. The 89-year- old father of a friend swears by this technique. He chews his food 100 times and has never had indigestion. While 100 times may be a bit much for most people, chewing your food very thoroughly, maybe two or three times as long as you normally do, may help to prevent frequent bouts of heartburn and acid reflux.

Dehydration

One of the most important things that we can do for our health, our digestion, our organs, and our bodies in general is to drink water. This is especially true for the elderly. As we get older, our kidneys work more slowly, and if you do not drink enough water, medications can build up in your system to an unhealthy level.

In addition, as you get older, your thirst mechanism, which tells you when you need water, often does not work as well. So, do not depend on feeling thirsty to alert you when to drink! Drink lots of water or other liquids, and eat lots of fruit, so you can stay hydrated, especially if you live in a warmer climate.

Be Your Own Sherlock Holmes

In this age of fragmented, cost-conscious health care, a doctor rarely knows the entire health care picture of each of his or her patients. Most doctors focus on their areas of expertise and hope that a patient's other doctors will do their parts in the other areas. Even general practitioners can have a hard time keeping track of all the ailments of every patient and the various treatments each patient has received for those ailments. And that does not even take into account all the information a patient "forgets", either intentionally or unintentionally, to tell the doctor. Therefore, you, or your health buddy, might want to channel Sherlock Holmes from time to time, especially when an ailment is puzzling or fails to respond to the standard treatments. Sherlock Holmes, the expert detective, is able to put together all the information (which may include changes in non-health care aspects of a patient's life), and deduce the answer to the health care mystery.

For example, I remember a health care mystery from back when I was a nurse in the hospital. A woman was admitted to the hospital because she was having chest pains. After several days of testing, she developed diarrhea, which became quite severe. Further diagnostic tests could not determine a cause for the diarrhea. As part of my job, I interviewed her about her diet to try to determine a cause. She said that since she had been in the hospital, she had not had much of an appetite, and the only food or drink she wanted was grape juice. Instead of the single glass of grape juice she had been used to drinking at home, she was drinking three or four glasses a day, which was causing her to have diarrhea. When she stopped drinking the grape juice, her diarrhea ceased, and she was able to go home (with medication for her heart).

Thus, it can helpful to be aware of even relatively minor changes in diet or routine, and to channel Sherlock Holmes when a health ailment is baffling!

Nine

Final Thoughts

The one idea I hope you take from this book is that a positive attitude can go a long way toward improving your life. Disability and infirmity often force us to navigate the fine line between acceptance (of limitations and situations) and resignation (giving up). In my experience, a positive attitude has helped me to accept the new limitations and situations that have occurred in my life, and to make my life as comfortable and enjoyable as I can despite them. I am always thinking of ways to make my life better, and then I try my best to implement them. If something is a problem, endless complaining is not the answer. Instead I either make changes to fix the problem, or accept the situation and move on. Life is too short for endless complaining or pity parties!

Speaking of parties, I strongly believe in having parties in my everyday life. Why wait for special occasions? At this time, I do not require 24-hour care, but I have wonderful paid companions that come for about 9 hours per day. They prepare food, do laundry, and take me to appointments and shopping, and help with other activities that I am unable to do on my own. Most important, however, when they walk into my home, it is party time, and we have fun! We also frequently invite my friends and neighbors over for parties to celebrate birthdays, non-birthdays, and any other reason or non-reason we can think of. This everyday fun is gives me a good quality of life. And I won't settle for less!

Appendix A

Example of Medical Log

3/1/10   Dr. T. Smith
Primary Care Physician
Annual Checkup

5/8/10   Broken Ankle
E.R. at Southside Hospital
Medications: Tylenol for pain
Instructions: Follow up w/ Physical
Therapy

8/2/10   Lab Work
Quest Diagnostics
SED rates and cholesterol

9/15/10   Dr. C. Owens
Cardiologist
EKG good

9/22/10   Dr. M. Jones
Dentist
X-rays
No cavities!

Appendix B

Example of Medication List

<u>Morning medications:</u>

Lisinopril – 20 mg – 1 tablet daily

Prilosec (Omeprazole) – 1 tablet daily

Centrum Silver for Women – 1 tablet daily

<u>Evening medications:</u>

Crestor – 5 mg – 1 tablet nightly

<u>Other medications:</u>

Tylenol – 250 mg – taken for pain as needed.

Appendix C

Example of Medical History

Name: Jane Doe
Address: 222 Mockingbird Lane,
Central City, FL 33112
Phone: 222-222-5555
Date of Birth: 7/18/1935
Blood Type: A positive

Primary Insurance: Blue Cross cc25252525
Secondary Insurance: None

Emergency Contact: John Doe
Phone: 222-5555

Previous Diagnoses:
Blood clot in left leg vein – 2/2010
Lumbar spinal fracture – 6/2008
Temporal Arteritis – 4/2007
Osteoporosis – 3/1996

Surgical History:
Appendectomy – 7/1972

Family History
Mother: Deceased of heart failure at age 89
Father: Deceased of lung cancer at age 72

Resources

The Boulevard – A Disability Resource Directory of Products and Services for the Physically Challenged, Elderly, Caregivers and Healthcare Professionals
www.blvd.com

Independent Living Aids, LLC – Independent Living Aids for Your Active Lifestyle
800-537-2118
www.independentliving.com

Maxi Aids – Products for Independent Living
800-522-6294
www.maxiaids.com

National Council on Disability
202-272-2004
www.ncd.gov

National Federation of the Blind
www.nfb.org

Sight Connection- Products for Living Well With Vision Loss
800-458-4888
www.sightconnection.com

Woodland Manufacturing – Customized alphabet letters for labeling items
www.woodlandmanufacturing.com

www.ingramcontent.com/pod-product-compliance
Lightning Source LLC
Chambersburg PA
CBHW070537290526
45790CB00002B/537